Paleo Slow Cooker Recipes

Easy, Nutritious Food the Whole Family Will Love

Contents

About the Book

     This book can be a helping guide to following the Paleolithic diet and using your crockpot to make it simple. Set it and forget it! You will find an introduction to the Paleo diet first. The recipes will start after that with breakfast, then stews and soups, main dish ideas and desserts. You will find the main dishes organized by meat type. All of the recipes can be easily made in the crockpot and are very nutritious and delicious. Happy slow cooking!

Introduction

The Paleolithic diet is more of a new lifestyle going back to basics. It is based on the principles of eating real food that is available in our natural environment. Science has been discovering that our bodies are not well adapted to the new foods that were introduced about 10-15,000 years ago. The diet focuses on nutrient dense, fresh foods including meats, fruits, vegetables, nuts, eggs and fish. If the food is processed, modified, refined or partial, it is not Paleo because it is not found naturally. One great thing about this diet is: It is easy to remember what foods you can eat. Just ask yourself if it is natural and ask where it came from.

The diet does not include bread, cereal or pasta which has shown to cause inflammation, weight gain and blood sugar problems, just to name a few. The Paleo diet does end up being lower carbohydrate because you are eating more fruits and vegetables. The diet reduces inflammation, increases energy levels, body performance and composition. You will consume higher fat content, sometimes higher calories and high protein contents and can still lose weight. Enjoy these recipes that share delicious ways to combine natural healthy foods into delicious recipes for your daily life. Don't forget the sweets too! Yes, nature included some nutrient rich indulgences.

Breakfast

Maple Butternut Squash

1 large butternut squash (peeled and cubed)

½ c. maple syrup

1 lemon (juice squeezed)

1 tsp. pumpkin pie spices

4 tbsp. butter

Turn the heat on the crockpot to high and add the butter. Allow it to melt then mix in the squash and syrup. Then squeeze the juice out of the lemon and add the spices. Combine well and cook for 4 hours on high heat,

Breakfast Pie

8 large eggs

2 c. spinach

1 lb. pork sausage

1 onion (chopped)

1 tbsp. garlic powder

2 tsp. basil

Salt to taste

Pepper to taste

8 oz. mushrooms (sliced)

2 zucchinis (chopped)

Coconut oil as needed

Cover the inside of the crockpot with coconut oil. Whisk the eggs together, chop up the sausage and prepare vegetables. Add everything together in the crockpot and mix. Cook for 7 hours on low. Slice into pieces and serve.

Breakfast Tacos

2 lbs. pork (boneless short ribs)

2 tbsp. maple syrup

2 tsp. garlic powder

Salt to taste

Place the pork in the crockpot and mix in maple syrup, garlic powder and salt. Once well combined cook on low for about 9 hours.

3 large eggs

½ c. coconut milk

2 tbsp. coconut flour

Salt to taste

Once the pork has cooked for 9 hours, remove it, shred it and pour some of the liquid onto it. Then mix together the eggs, milk, flour and salt. Mix until it is no longer lumpy. Then heat up a skillet over medium-high heat and add some butter or oil. Then pour some of the egg mixture into the skillet. Let it cook until lightly browned, then flip it and brown the other side. These should be about 5 inches in diameter. Repeat until the tortilla mixture is gone. Set aside

1 8 oz. can of green chilies

3 tbsp. hot sauce

Green onions to taste

6 bacon strips

Next add the bacon into the medium-high heated skillet. Brown on both sides. Remove and break into about inch wide pieces. Then mix together your green chilies and hot sauce and heat over medium heat for about 2 minutes. Then add in your bacon. Chop up the green onions. Now take a tortilla, add some pork, the chili bacon mixture and top with green onions. Then serve.

Breakfast Scramble

8 large eggs

1 yam

1 lb. pork sausage

1 large onion (yellow)

1 tbsp. garlic powder

2 tsp. basil (dried)

Salt to taste

Pepper to taste

Whisk together the eggs well. Shred the yam. Break up the sausage. Dice the onion. Then mix all ingredients together well. Grease the crockpot and add the mixture in. Let cook for about 7 hours on low, then use a spatula to cut out pieces and serve.

Maple Pork Breakfast

3 lbs. pork roast (shoulder)

2 c. blueberries

½ c. apple juice

¼ c. maple syrup

1 tsp. cinnamon

1 tsp. parsley

½ tsp. sage

¼ tsp. nutmeg

Salt to taste

Pepper to taste

5 bacon strips

Fresh parsley

Pour apple juice into the bottom of the crockpot and place the pork roast in. Then cover with the maple syrup and all of the seasonings. Lastly add in the blueberries and cook for about 9 hours on low heat. After 9 hours transfer the pork into a bowl and shred it with a fork, then add some of the juices to keep it moist. In a medium sized skillet cook the bacon strips until browned on both sides. Then drain them on a paper towel and cut into 1 inch pieces. Save the fat from the bacon. Split the bacon into two parts. Combine the first part with the shredded pork and make into patties. Fry the patties in the bacon fat for about 4 minutes on each side. Then top with bacon and parsley and serve.

Breakfast Cobbler

6 apples

½ c. coconut

½ c. milk (coconut)

½ c. raisins

Plenty of cinnamon

1 tbsp. vanilla

Salt to taste

Remove the cores and skin from the apples and chop them up. Cover the inside of your crockpot with coconut oil and then add in all ingredients. Mix together well and cook for 6 hours on low.

Egg Casserole

2 sweet potatoes

2 cloves of garlic

1 red onion

1 red bell pepper

1 tbsp. butter

12 large eggs

1 c. milk (coconut)

8 strips bacon

Red pepper flakes to taste

Salt to taste

Pepper to taste

Cover the inside of your crockpot with coconut oil. Chop up the onion and bell pepper. Grate the sweet potatoes and mince the garlic. Add butter to a medium skillet and add the red onions, garlic and bell pepper cooking them until they soften. Then remove and add the bacon strips and cook until brown on both sides. Then remove and crumble. Split the potato, bacon and onion mixture into three parts. Add 1 section of potatoes then onion mixture then bacon and repeat 3 times. Then whisk all of your eggs, milk, salt, pepper and red flakes and pour in crockpot over the layers. Cook for 8 hours on low heat then cut and serve.

Appetizers

Sweet Spice Nuts

2 c. mixed nuts of your choice

½ c. seeds

1 tbsp. maple syrup

½ tsp. salt

½ tsp. cayenne pepper

Coconut oil as needed

Cover the inside of the crockpot with coconut oil. Mix together the nuts, seeds and syrup and sprinkle in the salt and cayenne pepper to your liking. Mix so that the nuts and seeds are thoroughly covered and put in the crockpot for 20 minutes on high and then 1 and a half hours on low with the lid off. The nuts will have a nice glaze. Then let them cool on parchment paper and enjoy or refrigerate for later.

Cha Dan

12 large eggs

2 black tea bags

4 tbsp. salt

6 star anise

2 tbsp. cinnamon

1 tbsp. peppercorns

1 tsp. black pepper

7 c. water

Bring a large pot of water to a boil and add the eggs. Once hard boiled after about 10 minutes remove them and let them cool. Crack the shells but do no break them off of the egg. In a crockpot, combine the remaining ingredients and add the eggs back in then cover with 6 cups of water. Turn to low heat and cook for 30 minutes. Take the tea bags out and continue cooking for about 4 more hours. Then remove the eggs and let them cool off. Now remove the shells and serve.

Bacon Brussels sprouts

1 lb. of brussel sprouts (washed and trimmed)

1 tbsp. Dijon mustard

Salt to taste

Pepper to taste

2 tbsp. butter

6 oz. bacon

Start by heating a medium skillet over medium high heat and frying the bacon until browned on both sides. Transfer to a paper towel to drain and cool. Slice the bacon into about 1 inch ling pieces. Slice the brussel sprouts in half and add them to the crock pot along with the bacon, mustard, butter, salt and pepper. Mix well cook for 4 hours on low. Then serve.

Hot Wings

4 lbs. chicken (legs or wings)

¾ c. butter

½ c. hot sauce (Franks)

2/3 c. apple cider vinegar

¾ tsp. paprika

½ tsp. black pepper

Heat up your oven to broil and set the chicken in there for 5 minutes per side to get a crispy outer layer. In a small sauce pan add the butter and melt over low. Then combine with remaining ingredients. Transfer the chicken to the crockpot and cover them with the sauce. Then cook for 2 hours on high.

Chicken Rolls

4 chicken breasts

6 slices spiced ham

24 asparagus spears

3 cloves of garlic

Salt to taste

Pepper to taste

Start by pounding your chicken breasts flat with a mallet. The slice each breast in half. Next roll up 3 asparagus spears in each piece of chicken and roll it up. Then trim off excess asparagus. Roll the chicken up in a piece of ham and secure with a toothpick. Then cook for 4 hours in the crock pot.

Turkey and Veggie Balls

1 lb. ground turkey

2 large eggs

½ c. pine nuts

1 c. grated zucchini

1 c. chopped red onion

2 c. crushed tomatoes

6 oz. spinach leaves

In a large bowl whisk the eggs and combine with the zucchini and onions. Then mix in the turkey until thoroughly combined. Next pour half of the tomatoes into the crockpot. Top with half of the spinach. Then roll your turkey combination into 1 ½ inch balls and set on top of the spinach. Next add another layer of tomatoes, spinach then pine nuts. Cook on low for 6 hours then enjoy.

Cucumber and Pork Refreshers

5 lb. pork loin

3 c. mint

1 orange

2 limes

½ c. EVOO

2 garlic cloves

1 white onion

1 watermelon (seedless)

2 large cucumbers

Salt to taste

Pepper to taste

Combine the mint, juice from the orange, juice from the limes, EVOO and garlic in a food processor. Process well and pour into a container or bag. Season the pork to your liking with salt and pepper. Then add the pork into the mint mixture and let marinate overnight or for about 5 hours in the fridge. After it marinates, add the sliced onions to the crockpot base and top with the marinated pork. Cook for 5 hours on low. Slice the watermelon, pork and cucumber into ¼ of an inch pieces that are about 1 inch in length. Then stack them up and top with a mint leaf. Secure the stack with a toothpick and serve.

Pork Lettuce Wraps

3 lb. pork roast

6 chipotle peppers with adobe sauce

8 oz. pineapple with juice

1 white onion

½ c. orange juice

4 garlic cloves

1 tbsp. vinegar (apple cider)

1 tsp. dried oregano

1 tsp. cinnamon

1 tsp. dried cumin

Black pepper to taste

Salt to taste

Romaine Lettuce head

Salsa for garnish:

Pineapple

White onion

Cilantro

2 limes (juice)

First you will process the marinade in a food processor. Crush the pineapple, dice the onion and crush the garlic cloves. Combine together all ingredients except the pork and lettuce in the processor. Combine thoroughly and transfer to a container with the pork to marinate in the fridge overnight. Then add to the crockpot and cook for 6 hours on low. Then shred the meat with a fork and serve it on lettuce leaves. For salsa process the ingredients and spoon on top of the pork in the lettuce wrap.

Honey Mustard Ribs

Ribs:

3 tbsp. vinegar (balsamic)

3 tbsp. Worcestershire

2 tbsp. honey

3 tsp. mustard (brown)

1 tsp. hot sauce

1 c. chicken broth

1 piece ginger (about 1 inch)

1.5 lb. pork ribs

Glaze:

¼ c. mustard

2 tbsp. water

1 tbsp. honey

2 tsp. vinegar (apple cider)

1 tsp. tomato paste

1 tsp. soy sauce (gluten free)

Cayenne pepper to taste

Black pepper to taste

In a small bowl mix together the all ingredients in the ribs section except the ribs. Combine well. Then place the ribs in the crockpot and cover with the sauce. Cook for 7 hours on low. Then combine the glaze ingredients. Remove the ribs from the crockpot and brush the glaze onto them and serve. Delicious!

Chicken Shawarma Salad

3 lbs. chicken thighs (sliced)

2 yellow onions (sliced)

3 tbsp. olive oil

1 lemon (for juice)

3 cloves of garlic (mince)

1 tsp. allspice

1 tsp. salt

1 tsp. cumin

1 tsp. coriander

½ tsp. pepper

½ tsp. paprika

Combine all seasonings together in a small bowl. Cover chicken thighs and onions in olive oil and lemon juice then cover in the seasoning mixture. Refrigerate for 5 hours. Then add to the crockpot and cook on low for 6 hours. Then heat olive oil in a large skillet and brown the outside of each thigh piece. Set aside.

Salad:

Mixed Greens

Cucumber (slice)

Tomato (slice)

Parsley (chopped)

Top the mixed greens with the cucumber, tomato, parsley and chicken pieces. Drizzle with olive oil and some fresh squeezed lemon juice and serve.

Dinner Stews

Easy Beef and Cabbage Stew

2 lbs. sauerkraut

1 head of red cabbage

1.5 lbs. beef kielbasa (sliced into 1 inch slices)

Shred the cabbage and add to the crockpot along with the sauerkraut and kielbasa. Mix well and cook for 5 hours on low. Then enjoy!

Beef Plantain Stew

2.5 lbs. beef short ribs

6 medium plantains

3 c. collard greens (chopped)

3 c. water

1/3 c. paprika

1/4 c. garlic powder

3 tbsp. salt

3 tbsp. allspice

1 tsp. chili powder

1 tsp. cayenne pepper

In a large skillet sear the outside of the beef ribs. Transfer to a crockpot and add the remaining ingredients. Cook for 8 hours on low then serve.

Butternut Soup

6 c. butternut squash (cut into cubes)

14 oz. coconut milk

2 c. chicken stock

1 apple (peel, remove core and cut into cubes)

2 carrots (peel and slice)

1 tbsp. cinnamon

1 tbsp. nutmeg

Combine all the ingredients together in the crockpot and cook on low for 6 hours. Add soup into a blender and blend to desired consistency. Then serve it up.

Sausage and Kale Stew

12 oz. smoked sausage

8 oz. kale

1 large onion

4 carrots

3 potatoes

5 c. chicken broth

1 bay leaf

Black pepper to taste

Remove the stems from the kale and chop into bite size pieces. Chop up the onion. Peel and chop the potatoes. Chop the carrots into 1.2 inch pieces. Slice the sausage into ¼ inch slices. Heat a medium sized skillet over medium high heat with some olive oil and add the onions and sausage. Brown and transfer to crockpot with the rest of the ingredients. Cook on low for 6 hours and enjoy!

Chicken Enchilada Soup

2 lbs. chicken

1 onion (yellow)

1 bell pepper (green)

4 oz. jalapenos (chopped)

4 oz. green chilies

2 tbsp. coconut oil

14 oz. tomatoes diced

7 oz. tomato sauce

3 cloves of garlic

1 tbsp. cumin

1 tbsp. chili powder

2 tsp. oregano

Salt to taste

Pepper to taste

Cilantro

Avocado slices

Start by chopping up your onion, bell pepper, jalapenos, and green chilies. Then mince the garlic. Dice the tomatoes. Slice the avocado and chop up the cilantro. Then add everything into the crockpot and combine well. Set your crockpot to low and cook for about 9 hours.

Sweet Potato Soup

2 yams (diced)

1 yellow onion (1/2 diced)

14 oz. coconut milk

1 c. vegetable broth

2 minced cloves of garlic

1 tbsp. basil (dried)

Salt to taste

Pepper to taste

Mix all ingredients together in the crockpot and cook on high for 3 hours. After 3 hours use an immersion blender if you have one or transfer all into a blender. Blend until smooth and serve.

Beef Mushroom Soup

2 lbs. beef (meat for stew)

8 oz. sliced mushrooms

8 oz. shiitake mushrooms (whole)

8 oz. Portobello mushrooms (baby)

1 yam

4 cloves of garlic

1 c. pearl onions

1 c. beef broth

1/3 c. balsamic vinegar

2 tbsp. vinegar (red wine)

1 bay leaf

2 tbsp. onion powder

1 tbsp. rosemary (dried)

1 tsp. parsley

Salt to taste

Pepper to taste

Start by soaking the onions in water for 5 minutes and peeling off the skin. Then crush up the garlic cloves. Combine the garlic, onions and mushrooms in the crockpot. Then chop up your yam and add that along with the beef on top of the onions. Add the bay leaf, onion powder, rosemary, sage, parsley, salt and pepper. Then lastly add the vinegars and beef broth. Cook on low heat for about 7 hours

Tomato soup with Mussels

2 lbs. mussels

3 tbsp. olive oil

4 cloves of garlic

3 cloves of shallots

8 oz. mushrooms

30 oz. diced tomatoes

2 tbsp. oregano

½ tbsp. basil

Pinch of pepper

Pinch of paprika

Red chili flakes to taste

3/4 c. water

Over medium high heat, add the olive oil and sauté the mushrooms, shallots and garlic until lightly browned. Then combine the mixture with the remaining ingredients except for the mussels. Mix in crockpot and cook on low for 5 hours. Clean the mussels and add them to crockpot for 30 minutes on high, Throw away any mussels that have not opened up. Then serve and enjoy.

Hearty Beef Stew

3 lbs. beef (stew meat)

6 carrots (diced)

1 onion (diced)

1 c. apricots (dried and quartered)

½ c. raisins

5 cloves of garlic

1 tsp. cumin

1 tsp. paprika

½ tsp. cinnamon

Pinch of cayenne pepper

3 c. beef broth

In a large pan sear the outsides of your beef then add to the crockpot. Then add the onions to the skillet and sauté in coconut oil, when they start to turn translucent add minced garlic, cumin, paprika, cinnamon and cayenne pepper. Mix well and allow onions to absorb flavor. Transfer into the crockpot. Next add in the rest of your ingredients and mix up. Cook on low heat for about 9 hours. Then serve.

Dutch Beef Stew

2lbs. beef

4 tbsp. of butter

3 onions (diced)

2 tbsp. arrowroot

4 tbsp. tomato paste

2 c. beef broth

½ c. red wine

2 apples

2 t. molasses

1 tsp. rosemary

1 bay leaf

Salt to taste

Pepper to taste

In a large skillet over medium-high heat melt the butter and add the meat. Brown on all sides and transfer to crockpot. In the same pan add the onions and cook until softened. Peel the skin off of the apples and chop. Transfer to the crockpot and add the remaining ingredients. Mix together thoroughly and cook on low for 8 hours. Remove bay leaf.

Seafood Stew

28 oz. tomatoes and juice

8 oz. tomato sauce

1 onion

1 green pepper

1 c. white wine

1/3 c. olive oil

4 cloves of garlic

2 tbsp. parsley

1 tsp. dried thyme

2 tsp. dried basil

2 tsp. dried oregano

1 tsp. chili paste

Pinch of black pepper

Pinch of salt

Cayenne pepper to taste

1 lb. mussels, clams, white fish, scallops, cooked crab meat

Water

Chop the onion and green pepper and mince the garlic. Then combine with the tomatoes and all seasonings. Pour in crockpot and cook on low for 8 hours. Then add the seafood and cook on high for 30 minutes, remove closed clams and mussels and trash. Then serve.

Potato and Bacon Soup

8 potatoes (peeled and diced)

1 onion (chopped)

1 carrot (sliced)

2 cloves of garlic

3 ½ c. chicken stock

Cayenne pepper to taste

6 bacon strips (browned and broken into small pieces)

In a crockpot combine the potatoes, onion, carrots, minced garlic, chicken stock and cayenne pepper to your liking. Mix well and cook for 8 hours on low heat. Blend the soup to desired consistency and serve topped with bacon bits.

Pumpkin Chili

14.5 oz. pumpkin (process to smooth)

14.5 oz. tomatoes (chop)

1 green bell pepper (deseed and chop)

1 red bell pepper (deseed and chop)

1 white onion (chop)

3 cloves of garlic (mince)

1 lb. of ground turkey

1 tbsp. chili powder

Black pepper to taste

Cumin to taste

Salt to taste

½ c. water

In a large skillet heat some olive oil over medium high heat. Add the turkey to the skillet and sauté until browned. After about 10 minutes add in the tomatoes, onion, peppers and garlic and allow them to soften. Then transfer into the crockpot. Mix in all seasonings and water and cook for 6 hours on low.

Minestrone Soup

1 1/2 lb. ground sausage

2 tbsp. olive oil

1 sweet potato (chopped)

1 c. carrots (chopped)

2 stalks of celery (chopped)

2 zucchini (peeled and chopped)

2 small onions (chopped)

2 cloves of garlic (mince)

28 oz. vegetable broth

28 oz. diced tomatoes

1 c. spinach leaves (chop)

1 bay leaf

2 tsp. dried oregano

1 tsp. dried basil

1 tsp. dried parsley

Cayenne pepper to taste

1/4 tsp. salt

Oil the crock pot with olive oil. Mix together all the ingredients except for the sausage. Combine well and set to low heat. Two hours in cook the sausage in a large frying pan. Break it up and cook until thoroughly browned. Then add to the rest of ingredients, mix and cook for 6 more hours. Once the time is up, take out the bay leaf and serve.

Chicken and Black Bean Soup

15 oz. black beans (cooked)

3 ½ c. chicken broth

10 oz. tomatoes

2 oz. green chilies (chopped)

1 bell pepper (red chopped)

4 oz. green chilies (diced)

1 tbsp. cumin

1 tsp. chili powder

¼ tsp. dried oregano

2 chicken breasts

½ c. cilantro (chopped)

1 medium yellow onion (diced)

1 scallion (chopped)

2 limes (quartered)

1 avocado (slice)

Process half of the black beans in a food processor with half of the chicken broth. Transfer to the crockpot and mix the remaining beans and chicken broth in. Add remaining ingredients except for ...and cook for 7 hours on low. When it is done, break apart the chicken and adjust seasonings to taste and add in the scallion. Then let cook for 15 more minutes, then serve with lime quarters and slices of avocado.

Black Bean Soup

1 lb. black bean (raw)

1 red bell pepper (chopped)

1 yellow onion (chopped)

2 garlic cloves (mince)

2 bay leaves

Soup:

Splash of olive oil

1 yellow onion (processed)

½ c. parsley (chop)

1 pepper (red, minced)

2 carrots (shred)

5 garlic cloves (mince)

1 tbsp. vinegar (red wine)

1 tsp. dried cumin

1 tsp. dried oregano

Salt to taste

Pepper to taste

Soak the black beans overnight in a pot of water. Drain in the morning and pour into the crockpot, then cover with fresh water. Add the bay leaves, onions, bell pepper and garlic and mix with the beans. Cover and cook on low for 8 hours. After 5 hours add the carrots, pepper, garlic, red wine, oregano, cumin, vinegar and onion. Add salt and pepper to taste and cook for 3 more hours. When finished fish out the bay leaves and blend the soup until smooth. You can transfer it to a blender in portions or use an immersion blender. Then serve and top with cilantro and green onions.

Carrot and Ginger Soup

1 tbsp. butter

1 white onion (chop)

3 c. chicken broth

1 lb. baby carrots (peel)

1 tbsp. ginger

Salt to taste

Pepper to taste

2 tbsp. green onions (chopped)

In a small skillet, melt the butter and sauté onions. Transfer to the crockpot and combine with broth, carrots and ginger, Cook on low for 6 hours. Blend the soup with an immersion blender or regular blender in portions. Then serve.

Bison Soup

2 lbs. bison meat

2 yellow medium onions (slice)

5 carrots (peel them and slice)

1 green bell pepper (chopped)

3 celery stalks (chopped

2 jalapenos (chopped and deseeded)

28 oz. roasted tomatoes

8 oz. tomato sauce

Fresh cilantro

1 tbsp. dried oregano

Salt to taste

Pepper taste

After preparing the vegetables put them in the base of your crock pot then top with the bison and then all other ingredients. Cook for 7 hours on low.

Main Dishes

Beef

Chili on Rice

2 onions (yellow)

4 garlic cloves (mince)

2 bell peppers (green)

2 lb. beef (ground chuck)

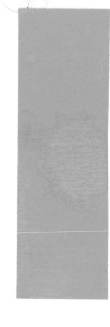

14 oz. tomatoes

4 oz. green chili

2 tsp. cumin

1 tbsp. oregano

1 tsp. cayenne

Black pepper to taste

Salt to taste

1 c. chicken broth

1 cauliflower head

In a medium pan heat some olive oil over medium high heat. Add the onions, garlic and peppers to the oil and cook until softened. Next add in beef and brown until the pink is gone. Add in everything else except the cauliflower to the crockpot and combine with the meat. Cook for 6 hours on low heat. Add the cauliflower to the food processor and blend until it is reduced to tiny pieces that look like rice. Put it in a bowl and heat for about 5 minutes. Sprinkle salt and pepper on the cauliflower and serve topped with chili.

Asian Style Roast

2 lb. beef roast

1 c. soy sauce gluten free

8 oz. beef broth

2 tbsp. salt

1 tbsp. onion (mince)

1 tbsp. garlic powder

1 tbsp. cilantro

Black pepper to taste

3 anise stars

4 c. water

Combine all ingredients together in the slow cooker and cook for 8 hours on low heat.

Stuffed Peppers

4 peppers (red, green, yellow orange bells)

1 lb. ground beef

½ head cauliflower

1 large onion (chopped)

1 carrot (chopped)

4 garlic cloves (mince)

6 oz. tomato paste

Salt to taste

Pepper to taste

¼ c. beef broth

Start by cutting the tops off of the bell peppers and clean out the insides. Then process the carrots, cauliflower, onion and garlic until very fine. Combine the processed veggies in a medium bowl with the beef and tomato sauce. Add salt and pepper to your likings. Then scoop the mixture to fill each bell pepper and put the tops back on. Then pour the beef stock into the crock pot and place the bell peppers in it. Cook for 8 hours on low.

Ropa Viejo

3 lb. steak (flank)

2 tbsp. coconut oil

¼ c. olive oil

1 tbsp. vinegar (white wine)

2 tbsp. salt

¼ c. cilantro

¼ c. parsley

2 garlic cloves (mince)

12 oz. tomato paste

1 green bell pepper (sliced)

1 red bell pepper (sliced)

1 yellow bell pepper (sliced)

1 tbsp. onion powder

1 tbsp. garlic powder

1 tbsp. dried oregano

1 tbsp. cumin

Slice the steak in strips of about 2 inches. Fry the steak in coconut oil over medium high heat in a skillet. Mix together all ingredients in the crock pot and cook for 6 hours on low heat. This comes out very flavorful, colorful and delicious! Enjoy!

Philly Cheesesteak

2 lb. ground beef

3 cloves of garlic

1 green bell pepper

1 red bell pepper

1 yellow onion

1 c. mushrooms

Black pepper to taste

1 tsp. cumin

½ tsp. oregano

Red pepper flakes to taste

Cayenne pepper to taste

½ lb. salami

Mix the pepper, cumin, oregano and red pepper flakes with the beef and add to a large skillet over medium high heat. Cook until the meat is browned thoroughly. Then transfer to crockpot and mix in chopped vegetables and chopped salami. Combine all ingredients well and cook on low heat for 5 hours.

Meatballs

2 lb. ground beef

2 lb. Italian sausage

4 large eggs

½ c. coconut milk

½ c. almond meal
½ parmesan cheese

4 garlic cloves

3 tbsp. basil

3 tbsp. oregano

Black pepper to taste

Salt to taste

Tomato Sauce:

2 can of tomatoes

1 can tomato sauce

4 garlic cloves minced

1 medium yellow onions (slice)

Pinch of basil, oregano, thyme, salt and pepper

Combine all meatball ingredients very thoroughly in a medium bowl and then use your hands to roll into balls. Then in another bowl combine the tomatoes, tomato sauce, garlic and seasonings. Now it is time to transfer it all into the crockpot. Layer onions, meatballs, sauce onions, meatballs, sauce. Cook on low for about 8 hours and enjoy.

Short Ribs

5 lb. beef short ribs

1750 ml red wine

2 tbsp. butter

1 onion (chopped)

3 celery (chopped)

3 carrots (chopped)

4 garlic cloves (chopped)

1 can tomato paste

3 c. beef broth

1 tbsp. thyme

1 tbsp. oregano

1 tbsp. rosemary

3 sweet potatoes (cubed)

Salt to taste

Pepper to taste

Season the ribs with salt, pepper, thyme, oregano and rosemary. Melt the butter in a large pot and brown the ribs on all sides. Then remove them and set them aside. Add in the onion, celery, carrots, and garlic and sauté until softened. Then add the tomato paste, wine and beef broth. Turn up the heat and add the ribs back in. Bring to a boil and transfer to the crock pot. Cook on low for 4 hours. Then add the potatoes and cook for 1 more hour. Then serve.

Shepherd's Pie
3 c. sweet potatoes

1 lb. ground beef

2 c. peas & carrots

1 medium onion

2 cloves of garlic

1 tbsp. herbs

½ c. beef broth

In a skillet over medium high heat sauté the chopped onion and minced garlic until browned, then add in the turkey and brown. Transfer to the crockpot with a bit of the fat and stir in the herbs, peas and carrots. Mash the sweet potatoes and put them on top of the meat and then pour the beef broth on top. Cook for 6 hours on low heat. Then turn up to high and cook an additional 30 minutes uncovered.

Mongolian Beef
2 lbs. beef (flank or round steak)

¼ c. beef broth

½ c. coconut aminos

5 cloves of garlic

6 green onions

2 carrots

2 tsp. vinegar (rice wine)

2 tsp. sesame oil

2 tsp. ginger

1 tsp. molasses

1 tbsp. almond butter

2 tbsp. raw honey

1 tbsp. red chili flakes

¼ tsp. pepper

Arrowroot powder as needed

Chop the green onions and crush the garlic. Combine everything together in the crockpot except the steak and mix well. Slice up your steak into thin pieces and cover in arrowroot powder. Set the meat slices on top of the mixture in the crockpot and cook on low for about 4 hours.

Italian Style Beef Roast

3 lb. beef roast (boneless)

1 large onion

14 oz. diced tomatoes

5 cloves of garlic

1 tbsp. oregano

1 tsp. rosemary

1 tsp. parsley

½ c. red wine

3 tbsp. olive oil

In a large skillet heat up the olive oil and brown the beef meat on all the sides. Once browned on all sides transfer to the crockpot. Then dice the onion and mince the garlic and cook until they soften. Then add the tomatoes, oregano, rosemary and parsley for 5-10 minutes. Then transfer the sauce into the crockpot and mix in with the beef. Then pour the wine on top of everything. Cook for about 8 hours on low then slice and serve.

Marinated Spare Ribs

5 lbs. short ribs (beef)

1 lime

2 tbsp. vinegar (white wine)

1 tbsp. honey

1 tbsp. sesame oil

2 tbsp. ginger

1 tsp. hot sauce

2 tsp. sesame seeds

Salt to taste

Pepper to taste

You will need a dish the ribs can fit in. In a medium bowl combine juice from the lime, vinegar, honey, sesame oil, ginger freshly grated, hot sauce, sesame seeds, salt and pepper. Mix well. Pour over the ribs in the dish and cover. Place in the refrigerator for 24 hours. Then transfer to the crockpot for 7 hours on low. Come back and enjoy!

Chicken

Salsa Verde Chicken Tenders

1 ½ lb. chicken tenders

¼ tsp. garlic powder

1/8 tsp. dried oregano

1/8 tsp. cumin

Salt to taste

8 oz. chopped tomatillos

4 oz. jalapenos chopped

4 oz. green chilies chopped

Process the tomatillos, jalapenos and green chilies in the food processor and set aside. Combine the seasonings and pat the chicken tenders with it. Put in your crockpot and cover with tomatillo mixture. Then cook for 4 hours on low.

Sticky Chicken

1 chicken

2 tsp. salt

1 tsp. cayenne pepper

1 tsp. paprika

2 tsp. garlic powder

1 tsp. thyme

½ tsp. black pepper

1 tsp. rosemary

1 medium yellow onion

In a small bowl mx together all the seasonings. Chop up the onion and layer it on the bottom of the crockpot. Then rub the seasoning mixture to cover the chicken completely. Place the chicken on top of the onions and cook on low for 8 hours. Then remove meat from the carcass and serve.

Herb Whole Chicken

4 lb. chicken

Olive oil

Thyme to taste

Rosemary to taste

Salt to taste

Pepper to taste

Place the chicken in the crockpot and cover in olive oil, spreading it to cover the whole chicken. Sprinkle salt, pepper, rosemary and thyme all over chicken and rub to cover entire bird. Cook for 8 hours on low. Then serve.

Cashew Chicken

2 lbs. chicken thighs

1 tbsp. raw honey

1 clove of garlic

Coconut oil as needed

½ tsp. ginger

2 c. broccoli

1 c. carrots

1 c. cashews

1 c. cilantro

¼ c. soy sauce (gluten free)

2 tbsp. vinegar (red wine)

Cover the inside of your crockpot in coconut oil so nothing sticks. Then mix soy sauce, grated ginger, garlic, honey and vinegar together and pour into crockpot. Add the chicken pieces Cook for 7 hours on low then add sliced carrots and broccoli for 1 more hour. Serve topped with cashews and chopped cilantro. .

Chicken Bacon Meatloaf

2 lbs. ground chicken

2 large eggs (whisked)

4 oz. bacon (browned and crumbled)

1 white onion (small and diced)

4 chives (chop)

2 celery stalks (chop thinly)

2 tsp. oregano

Black pepper to taste

Salt to taste

1 tsp. thyme

2 tsp. paprika

2 tsp. garlic powder

Sauce:

¼ c. tomato sauce

3 tbsp. mustard

2 tsp. paprika

2 tsp. garlic powder

1 tsp. vinegar (apple cider)

This recipe is very simple. After your bacon is browned and crumbled, get a large mixing bowl. Combine all ingredients for the meatloaf together and mix thoroughly. Form a loaf and place it in the crockpot. Next mix together all the ingredients for the sauce and cover the meatloaf with it. Cook for 5 hours on low then slice and serve.

Chicken Cacciatora

1 lb. boneless skinless chicken breast

3 tbsp. olive oil

1 green bell pepper

1 red bell pepper

1 yellow bell pepper

1 celery stalk

3 cloves of garlic

1 c. Tomatoes

1 white onion

Start by preparing the bell peppers by removing the stems and cleaning out the seeds. Then cut into slices. Next chop the tomatoes and celery stalk. Slice the onion and mince 2 of the garlic cloves. Combine the chicken, olive oil, sliced bell peppers, celery, garlic, and onion in the crock pot and combine thoroughly. Then add the tomatoes to the top. Cook for 8 hours on low heat.

BBQ Bacon Chicken

4 boneless, skinless chicken breast

8 pieces of bacon

¾ c. BBQ sauce

1 lemon

2 apples

Wrap each chicken breast in two pieces of bacon and secure with toothpicks. In a small bowl combine BBQ sauce with juice from the lemon and peeled and chopped apples. Place the chicken in the crockpot and cover with the BBQ sauce mixture. Cook for 8 hours on low heat. Serve and Enjoy!

Chinese Orange Chicken

2 lbs. chicken (thighs)

5 tbsp. tomato paste

1/8 c. orange juice

4 tbsp. coconut aminos

3 tbsp. honey

1 tsp. sesame oil

2 cloves of garlic

½ inch of ginger

½ tsp. rice vinegar

½ tsp. chili paste

2 tsp. arrowroot powder

Salt to taste

Pepper to taste

Mix together the tomato paste, orange juice, coconut aminos, honey, sesame oil, minced garlic, ginger, rice vinegar, salt and pepper and mix well. Add the chicken to the bottom of the crockpot and cover in marinade. Cook on low for 8 hours. Then remove thighs and add arrowroot powder and cook for 15 more minutes. Pour sauce on top of chicken and serve.

Indian Style Butter Chicken

3 lbs. boneless chicken thighs

1 large onion (chopped)

6 cloves of garlic

5 tbsp. of butter

2 tsp. curry powder

¼ tsp. cayenne pepper

Pinch of ginger

14.5 oz. coconut milk

6 oz. tomato paste

1 lemon (juice from it)

3 tsp. garam masala

Heat a medium skillet over medium high with olive oil. Mince the garlic and combine it with the onion and sauté until softened. Transfer to the crockpot and add the remaining ingredients including chicken. Mix well and cook on low for 8 hours.

Brazilian Chicken

2 lbs. chicken breasts

1 c. canned coconut milk

1 c. chicken broth

2 tbsp. tomato paste

3 garlic cloves

1 tbsp. ginger

5 tbsp. curry powder

2 bell peppers

1 onion (yellow)

Salt to taste

Pepper to taste

Red pepper to taste (flakes)

1 avocado

Combine all ingredients except the chicken and broth and mix well in the crockpot. After it is well combined add your chicken in and pour the chicken broth on top. Cook on low for about 7 hours. Serve in a bowl with sliced avocado on top.

Mushroom Chicken

2 lbs. boneless chicken thighs

2 tbsp. butter

1 medium onion

8 oz. mushrooms

1 tbsp. sage

1 tbsp. thyme

½ tarragon leaves

Take the mushrooms and slice them up. Then in a medium sized skillet add the 2 tbsp. of butter and melt it. Then dice up the onion and add to the skillet. Transfer the onions and butter to the crock pot, top with the chicken thighs, then add the seasonings and sliced mushrooms. Cook on low for 8 hours.

Balsamic Chicken

2 lb. chicken (thighs)

½ c. balsamic vinegar

5 cloves of garlic

2 tsp. oregano

2 tsp. parsley

Pepper to taste

12 oz. spinach leaves

Place the chicken thighs in the crockpot. In a medium bowl combine the vinegar, mince the garlic and add, oregano, parsley and pepper. Allow to cook on low heat for 6 hours. Then add spinach and cook for an additional 15 minutes then mix and serve.

Pork

Sweet Pulled Pork

5 lb. pork shoulder (I recommend with the bone)

1/8 c. brandy

2 tsp. salt

1 tsp. of cinnamon

1 tsp. dried ginger

1 tsp. nutmeg

Black pepper to taste

½ tsp. of dry mustard, onion and garlic powder

1/8 c. water

Mix together the salt, cinnamon, ginger, nutmeg, pepper, mustard, onion powder and garlic powder in a small bowl. Then cover each pork shoulder with the rub as thoroughly as you can. Fill the crockpot with 1/8 c. water and brandy and add the pork in. Cook for 7 hours on low.

Squash Lasagna

1 butternut squash (peel and cube)

1 zucchini (peel and cube)

1 white onion (chop)

1 lb. spicy Italian sausage

15 oz. tomato sauce

1 ½ tbsp. oregano

1 tbsp. basil

½ tbsp. paprika

Black pepper to taste

Salt to taste

¼ c. olive oil

1 red pepper (roasted)

Add a splash of olive oil to a large skillet over medium heat. Add the chopped onions and sausage and sauté until thoroughly cooked. Combine the olive oil, spices, pepper and tomato sauce in a food processor and process them throughout. Add the tomato mixture to the sausage once the sausage has cooked through. Now layer in the crockpot sauce, squash, sauce, squash, and sauce. Then cook for 4 hours on low heat.

Pork Fried Rice

1 cauliflower

1 lb. pork (boneless spare ribs)

2 tbsp. coconut oil

2 tsp. chili pepper

2 tsp. fresh ginger (mince)

4 garlic cloves (mince)

4 c. shredded cabbage

1 c. bean sprouts

½ c. green onions diced

1 large onion chopped

4 tbsp. gluten free soy sauce

4 tbsp. fish sauce

2 tbsp. chili paste

8 tbsp. water

4 large eggs

In a medium skillet add coconut oil and brown the ribs on all sides. Using a cheese grater, grate up the cauliflower thoroughly. Coat the crockpot in coconut oil and combine the ribs with the minced garlic, chili powder and ginger. Mix well. Stir in the soy and fish sauce and onions and cook on low for 6 hours. When finished mix in the cauliflower, cabbage, bean sprouts, scallions and water. Let cook for about 10 minutes more. Transfer to a large pot over high heat and cook until all the extra liquid has evaporated. Remove the pot from the heat and add the eggs stirring rapidly to incorporate them into the rice. Top with scallions and more uncooked bean sprouts and enjoy!

Apple Cinnamon Pork
2 pork chops (with the bone)

2 medium apples

1 yellow onion

1 red onion

4 tbsp. coconut oil

2 tbsp. raw honey

2 tsp. cinnamon

1 tsp. mustard powder

Salt to taste

Pepper to taste

Thinly slice the onions and apples. In a medium size skillet add 2 tbsp. of coconut oil and add the onions. In another skillet add 2 tbsp. of coconut oil and add the apples. Cook, stirring occasionally until they soften then add 1 tbsp. of honey, cinnamon and salt to each. Then combine the apples into the onions Let them caramelize over low heat. Transfer the apple onion mixture into the crockpot over low. Season the pork chops with all seasonings. Sear the outside of the pork chops in the pan you cooked the onions and apples in then transfer to the crockpot and cook on low for 5 hours.

Hawaiian Plate Meal
3 lb. pork (bone-in shoulder)

3 cloves of garlic

1 onion (yellow)

1 tsp. garlic powder

Pinch of salt

2 pieces of lettuce (romaine, chopped)

1 bell pepper (I prefer red)

4 oz. sliced mushrooms

2 c. pineapple

½ c. pepperoni

2 tbsp. butter

You will start with the crockpot. Cut up the yellow onion into slices and place at the bottom of the crockpot. Mince the garlic and add on top of the onions. Then add the pork on top. Add garlic powder and sprinkle with salt throughout. Then cook this on low heat for about 9 hours. After 9 hours use a fork to separate the meat. Next add a sauté pan to medium heat. Melt the butter and soften the mushrooms and more salt. Chop the bell pepper, pineapple and pepperoni then combine with the mushrooms and lettuce. Serve a scoop of pork with the combined salad.

Curry Pork
2 lbs. pork chops (boneless)

2 onions

4 garlic cloves

1 tbsp. fish sauce

1 tbsp. coconut amino

1 tbsp. turmeric (ground)

2 tsp. paprika

1 winter squash

Chop up the onion, squash and mince the garlic. In a small bowl combine the fish sauce, paprika, garlic, coconut aminos and turmeric. Cover the pork chops in this sauce and lay them at the bottom of the crockpot. Then layer the sliced onions over the pork. Then on top layer the chopped squash. Then cook on low for 7 hours and enjoy.

Pineapple Pork Ribs
2 lbs. pork ribs (Trim fat)

1 pineapple (cut into cubes of 1 inch)

1 tbsp. paprika

2 tbsp. mustard

1 tbsp. honey

In a small bowl combine the mustard, paprika and honey together and mix well. Lather the ribs in the mixture and transfer to the crockpot. Cover with pineapple and cook for 5 hours on low.

Other Meats

Fall off the bone Lamb Ribs

2 lbs. ribs of lamb

4 garlic cloves (minced)

1 yellow onion

2 tbsp. curry powder

3 tbsp. butter

Melt 1 tbsp. of butter in a medium-large skillet and sear the outside of each rib for a few minutes. Then slice the onion and mix it with the remaining 2 tbsp. of butter, curry powder and garlic and add to the crockpot with the ribs. Mix well and cook for 8 hours n low.

Fish Curry

1 lb. tilapia

13.5 oz. coconut cream

2 c. fish broth

2 carrots

3 celery stalks

2 tomatoes

2 tbsp. curry powder

1 tsp. turmeric

1 tsp. ginger

¼ c. cilantro

3 cloves of garlic (mince)

Salt to taste

Start by cutting the fish into 2 inch pieces. Then chop up the carrots, celery, cilantro and tomatoes. Add the carrots to a pot of boiling water and allow them to soften. Then add the remaining ingredients except the fish into the crockpot and cook on low for 6 hours. Add the fish and cook for 20-30 more minutes until the fish easily flakes.

Honey Mustard Salmon

2 salmon filets

3 tbsp. raw honey

2 tbsp. olive oil

1 tsp. Dijon mustard

1 tsp. ginger (ground)

Pinch of red pepper flakes

Combine in a small bowl honey, oil, mustard, ginger and flakes. Mix well. Place the salmon in parchment paper and cover the filets in the glaze. Place in the crockpot and cook for 2 hours on low heat.

Desserts

Chocolate Sweet Potato Dip

5 apples

3 sweet potato

¼ c. chocolate powder

¼ c. cinnamon

1 tbsp. ginger

1 tbsp. nutmeg

½ tsp. cloves

Peel and chop the apples and potatoes. Then combine them and the other ingredients into the crockpot. Cook on low for 10 hours then blend together. Goes great with apple pie.

Banana Dessert

4 medium bananas (cut into ¼ inch slices)

1 tbsp. coconut oil

1 lemon

3 tbsp. honey

Cinnamon to taste

Nutmeg to taste

In a small sauce pan combine the juice from a lemon, honey, coconut oil, nutmeg and cinnamon together. Heat over low-medium until it all melts and combines together. Combine this glaze with the bananas in the crockpot on low. Cook for about 2 hours, check after 1 and a half. Then enjoy.

Sweet Potato Treats

2 sweet potatoes (grated)

2 tbsp. coconut oil

½ tsp. cinnamon

Add coconut oil to crockpot. Spread throughout pan. Add the grated potatoes let cook for 3 hours on medium. Cover in cinnamon and serve.

Stuffed Apple Treats

4 apples (green)

½ c. coconut butter

¼ c. peanut butter

2 tbsp. cinnamon

½ tsp. nutmeg

Salt to taste

4 tbsp. shredded coconut (unsweetened)

1 c. water

Take the apples and remove the cored from the top. Leave the bottom of the apple intact so you can stuff the hollowed out core. Combine the butters and seasonings together well. Then stuff each apple with the mixture and top with coconut and sprinkle more cinnamon. Then transfer the apples into the crockpot, add the water, and cook for 3 hours on low heat. These will be softened and delicious.

Fudge

5 c. chocolate chips

1 c. coconut milk

½ c. honey

¼ tsp. salt

2 tsp. vanilla

Coconut oil

Pour the coconut milk into a bowl and stir until the consistency is even. Cover your crock pot with coconut oil. Then pour the coconut milk into the crockpot with the chocolate chips, honey and salt. Cook on high heat for 2 hours then add the vanilla in. Unplug the crock pot and leave uncovered to set for 3 hours. Then stir for about 10 minutes after the 3 hours is up. Transfer to an oiled container and refrigerate for about 10 hours. Then cut into squares and serve.

Honey Glazed Pears

4 pears

2/3 c. honey

1 tbsp. water

Nutmeg to taste

Ginger to taste

1 tbsp. arrowroot powder

2 tbsp. orange juice

Remove the cores of the pears from the bottom leaving the top intact. Place the pears in the crockpot. Then in a medium bowl mix together the ginger, honey and water and pour on top of the pears. Cook for 3 hours on high heat. Take the pears out after the 3 hours and add in the orange juice and arrowroot powder. Turn up the crockpot to high and cook for about 15 more minutes. Pour over the pears and enjoy.

Spiced Apples and Sweet Potatoes

6 small sweet potatoes

2 apples

2 tbsp. butter

Cayenne pepper to taste

Cinnamon to taste

Pinch of cumin

Pinch of salt

Peel the potatoes and apples. Remove the core of the apples. Slice both into ¼ inch slices and mix together. Transfer to the crockpot and mix in the cinnamon, cumin, salt and cayenne pepper. Mix well and add the butter. Cook for 6 hours on low heat. Then serve.

Pumpkin and Apple Butter

6 apples (peel, core and slice)

½ c. pumpkin (pureed)

½ c. coconut milk

½ c. pecans (processed)

1 tbsp. vanilla

½ tbsp. cinnamon

1 tsp. nutmeg

Cloves to taste (optional)

In a medium bowl mix together all ingredients except apples thoroughly. Add the apples to the crockpot and cover with pumpkin mixture. Cook for 6 hours on low then blend and serve with slices of raw apples and cinnamon sprinkled on top.

Apples, Dates and More

8 apples (peeled, cored and sliced)

1 c. dates

1 c. pecans

1 c. cherries

1 tbsp. cinnamon

1 tsp. pumpkin spice

½ tsp. nutmeg

¼ c. coconut oil

¼ c. honey

½ c. water

Chop the dates and process the pecans into pieces. Add to the crockpot with cherries and apples. Then mix in cinnamon, pumpkin spice, nutmeg and water. Mix together. The in a small sauce pan melt the honey and coconut oil then mix that into the crockpot too. Cook for 6 hours on low or 3 hours on high. Enjoy!

Brownies

½ c. almond butter

¼ c. raw honey

1/8 c. cocoa powder

1 tsp. vanilla

1 large egg

Salt to taste

¼ tsp. baking soda

Ground ginger to taste

In a medium bowl whisk the egg then combine with almond butter. Then mix in the honey, vanilla, salt, baking soda and ginger. Cover the inside of your crockpot with coconut oil then pour the brownie mix in. Cook for 1 ½ hours on high heat. Then cut and serve.

Honey Walnuts

3 tbsp. butter

¼ c. raw honey

1 tsp. vanilla

½ tsp. pumpkin pie spices

2 c. raw walnuts

Set your crockpot to high heat and add the butter so it can melt. Then add the honey and allow it to melt. Then mix in the vanilla, spices and walnuts. Mix everything together so that the walnuts are well coated. Cook for 1 and a half hours on high heat. Stir after each 30 minutes. Then enjoy. They are great refrigerated.

Made in the USA
Lexington, KY
08 March 2014